CW00519414

Mastering Intermittent Fasting For Women Over 50

An Easy And Understandable Guide To Fast And Easy Weight Loss, Burn Fat And Slow Aging Through Metabolic Process Of Autophagy, Increase Energy And Improve Your Life Quality

Anna Evans

© Copyright 2021 - All rights reserved.

The content contained within this book may not be reproduced, duplicated or transmitted without direct written permission from the author or the publisher.

Under no circumstances will any blame or legal responsibility be held against the publisher, or author, for any damages, reparation, or monetary loss due to the information contained within this book. Either directly or indirectly.

Legal Notice:

This book is copyright protected. This book is only for personal use. You cannot amend, distribute, sell, use, quote or paraphrase any part, or the content within this book, without the consent of the author or publisher.

Disclaimer Notice:

Please note the information contained within this document is for educational and entertainment purposes only. All effort has been executed to present accurate, up to date, and reliable, complete information. No warranties of any kind are declared or implied. Readers acknowledge that the author is not engaging in the rendering of legal, financial, medical or professional advice. The content within this book has been derived from various sources. Please consult a licensed professional before attempting any techniques outlined in this book.

By reading this document, the reader agrees that under no circumstances is the author responsible for any losses, direct or indirect, which are incurred as a result of the use of information contained within this document, including, but not limited to, errors, omissions, or inaccuracies.

Table Of Contents

INTRODUCTION

You may have heard about Intermittent Fasting from your friends, or maybe some random talk show mentioned it as some fat loss miracle. You've overheard some women at the gym bringing it up during their chat about carb-cycling and protein shakes, but what is it? The name says it all. Intermittent-periods; fasting—being without food. What's so special about periods without food? Every time I say the word fasting to my relatives, they get this big fearful look on their faces as if I am starving myself and could die at any moment! Fortunately, you won't be starving yourself. It's not one of those fasts that last 30 days and have you drinking lemonade and spices.

CHAPTER 1. HISTORY OF INTERMITTENT FASTING

When you feel the need to lose weight and cutting down your calories, you will find intermittent fasting the best way for sure. There are many ways by which you can reduce weight, but intermittent fasting or periodic fasting has many benefits apart from weight loss. Eating healthy, cutting down calories that are eating in a caloric deficit, and doing workouts will reduce weight. Here comes the question of how the idea of intermittent fasting came into being and who discovered it?

Fasting is an ancient ritual, which has been followed over the centuries by many cultures and religions. It is important to understand that fasting and starvation are two different things and shouldn't be mixed up. Starvation is a term used when the person has no idea about the availability of the meal, and there is a shortage of resources while fasting is avoiding the meals intentionally and the food is available.

Periodic fasting was used not just to cure the illnesses in ancient Egypt and Greece but also to prevent many diseases. Intermittent fasting was highly common in the middle Ages as people sought to enjoy its benefits. It was seen that intermittent fasting not only helps in reducing weight but also decreases insulin resistance. It is also used for the prevention of many diseases.

Intermittent fasting is the most common debate these days, so scientists are busy collecting intermittent fasting data. Studies conducted by Harvard have stated that fasting improves health, and those who practice intermittent fasting there are chances of increased life expectancy. This is quite obvious healthy individuals will survive longer because they will be physically active, and their body will be in the best state of health.

Intermittent fasting is both physical and religiously related. Many people practice intermittent fasting as part of their religion. Like Muslims, they fast in the holy month of Ramadan; Hindus observe different types of fasting according to their religion. Judaism has several common behaviors that include Yom Kippur, the truth of some. During the political times by a very famous leader Mahatma Gandhi at India's time of independence, Fasting was also observed.

In addition to controlling blood sugar, eating just one meal a day brings more benefits: reducing waist size and increasing muscle through the hormone HGH. Assuming the individual does not ingest non-protein foods, lowering blood pressure, improving lipid profile through lower LDL and higher HDL, reduced CRP or inflation, sound, even earlier, more significant over time as in any case, etc.

The concept of intermittent fasting has evolved with time. Starting from the point where it was considered starvation or due to insufficient sources, people used to stay hungry for a more extended period, the term fasting was identified. The definition of intermittent fasting has been changed from a period of fasting for hours or eating only one meal.

What Is Intermittent Fasting?

Intermittent fasting is described as an eating method that hovers between eating and fasting on a planned schedule. Several researchers have shown that this fasting method is very efficient for weight control and control of various kinds of diseases.

While several other diets focus on what you should eat, intermittent fasting focuses on what time to eat. Intermittent fasting restricts your eating plan to a specified period of the day, which, when followed, will make you lose weight, burn belly fat, and live a healthy life. There are several ways of doing intermittent fasting; yours is to study yourself and see the one that aligns with your health status and works best for you, then keep to it.

How Does Intermittent Fasting Work?

Even though there are several intermittent methods, the main routine of practicing all of them is to choose a pre-arranged period when you will eat and fast daily. An example is eating for 8 hours a day and fast for 16 hours, and you can also eat for five days of the weak and fast for the other two days (although both fasting days must not follow each other).

Intermittent fasting is different from the usual eating method because by eating three times a day together with snacks and not engaging in exercise, then you are only building your calories every time and not burning the fats storing in your body.

CHAPTER 2. BENEFITS OF INTERMITTENT FASTING FOR WOMEN OVER AGE 50

There are numerous benefits intermittent fasting has on the body of all humans and across all age groups. But in the course of this study, we are restricting our scope to women over 50. Some of these benefits are as follows:

Reduction in the Risk of Cancer

Intermittent fasting, which could also be referred to as mild caloric restriction, is very effective in the slowing down of fast-growing tumors that could lead to cancer.

Rous and Moreschi first discovered this benefit, and since then, it has gained wide recognition in the medical society. Restricting one's calorie intake also helps to boost the sensitivity of cancerous tumors to irradiation and chemotherapy.

Another benefit of intermittent fasting on women over 50 is the impairment of cancerous cells' metabolic process. This would make less energy available in the cell to function and most likely harm other cells.

Aside from that benefit, it serves to slow down, and if possible, shut down tumors, and it could help weaken them before treatments.

There is an action on transcription that boosts the effects of intermittent fasting against cancer. So, what is transcription? This is the process of copying information located in strands of DNA into molecular messengers called RNA.

The process is made possible by an enzyme known as RNA polymerase and many accessories of protein, which are classified as transcription factors. Some of these proteins include the forkhead box transcription factor (FOXO).

All the proteins play key roles in the process of metabolism, stress resistance, apoptosis (the programming process of cell death) as well as cellular proliferation (the process of cell growth).

Therefore, when this FOXO is activated during intermittent fasting, we could expect to see increased protection against carcinogenesis or tumorigenesis (the formation of cancer) and even the death of cancerous cells.

Another effect of FOXO's activation is increasing normal cells' resistance ability against stress, which could positively enhance the cells' longevity (and hence organisms).

Intermittent fasting may also play a key role in preventing cancer recurrence in women who had already been treated for cancer. Most times, these recurrences become more severe. Some cases of recurrence include stage IV breast cancer having a metastatic recurrence.

A study shows that women who carry out intermittent fasting exercise are less vulnerable to cancer recurrence (with a percentage of less than 36%). Intermittent fasting limits the amount of food that enters the body and reduces the amount of energy available to the cell.

Cells that are engaged in frequent restriction of Calories are known to less likely to develop changes that could lead to cancer. All these are owed to the positive and therapeutic effects of intermittent fasting on the cell and the immune system.

Reduces Cardiovascular Disease

Cardiovascular diseases (CVD) are known to have a very high mortality rate in women. Some of this CVD include; atherosclerotic cardiovascular disease (ASCVD), acute coronary syndrome (ACS), coronary artery disease (CAD), ischemic heart disease (IHD), etc.

Women above 50 have a higher chance of developing CVD, and although CVD affects both men and women, some risk factors increase the chances in women. These factors can be divided into two categories; modifiable and unmodifiable factors.

Among the unmodifiable factors are age, genetics, and gender. While the modifiable factors include hypertension, smoking, lack of physical exercise, obesity, poor diet, lipid metabolism disorder, diabetes, etc. Diabetes in women tends to increase the chances of a subtle heart attack without their knowledge.

Uncontrolled weight gain is the primary cause of obesity, which could lead to health disorders like diabetes, which increases the chances of developing CVD. Intermittent fasting has a great role it plays in insulin reduction, balancing heart rate, balancing high and low-density lipoprotein

Cholesterol (HDL and LDL). Also, it affects glucose levels as well as triglycerides, oxidative stress, and systemic inflammation.

Intermittent fasting boosts parasympathetic tone, which increases the variability of the heart rate. It does not only promote cardio-protection in overweight persons by enhancing weight loss; it works just as effectively in normal-weight individuals.

In other, for these positive changes to be lasting, one must continuously practice intermittently fasting, and the pattern or type of IF could depend on the preference of the individual.

Slows Down Aging Process

This is another benefit of intermittent fasting, and not until very recent years, the focus of intermittent fasting was to increase life span. This is because intermittent fasting was found to boost the body's general health and rejuvenate the body. The natural or even the induced aging process of the entire body is slowed down by doing this.

So, for women at 50 who, due to child-bearing and menopause, tend to age quicker than men, they can rely on strict adherence to intermittent fasting to slow down this process. The level of the effects of intermittent fasting varies from individual to individual.

However, its success is largely dependent on sex, age, genetic makeup, diet, environment, and other factors. Studies have shown that individuals who started intermittent fasting at a very young age have an increased lifespan (up to about 45%).

Individuals following a type of intermittent fasting experience strictly have a huge decrease in developing disorders that would be detrimental to their health. Hypertension, inflammation, obesity, dyslipidemia, and others, are lessened as a result of intermittent fasting. In fact, intermittent fasting is believed to have greater effects, which cannot be ascribed to only the reduction of calories.

Intermittent Fasting for Better Mental and Memory Performance

Intermittent fasting also enhances cognitive function and is very useful for boosting your brainpower. There are several factors of intermittent fasting, which can support this claim. First of all, it boosts the level of brain-derived neurotrophic factor (also known as BDNF), which is a protein in your brain that can interact with the parts of your brain responsible for controlling cognitive and memory functions as well as learning. BDNF can even protect and stimulate the growth of new brain cells.

Increase Physical Energy

This process influences not only your brain but also your digestive system. By setting a small feeding window and a larger fasting period, you will encourage the proper digestion of food. This leads to a proportional and healthy daily intake of food and calories. The more you get used to this process, the less you will experience hunger. If you are worried about slowing your metabolism, think again! Intermittent fasting enhances your metabolism; it makes metabolism more flexible, as the body now can run on glucose or fats for energy in a very effective way. In other words, intermittent fasting leads to better metabolism.

Oxygen use during exercise is a crucial part of the success of your training. You simply can't have performance without adjusting your breathing habits during workouts. VO2 max represents the maximum amount of oxygen your body can use per minute or kilogram of body weight. In popular terms, VO2 max is also referred to as "wind." The more oxygen you use, the better you will be able to perform. Top athletes can have twice the VO2 level of those without any training. A study focused on the VO2 levels of a fasted group (they just skipped breakfast) and a non-fasted group (they had breakfast an hour before). For both groups, the VO2 level was at 3.5 L/min at the beginning, and after the study, the level showed a significant increase of "wind" for the fasting group (9.7%), compared to just a 2.5% increase in the case of those with breakfast.

<u>Increase Longevity</u>

Autophagy is essential for the longevity of the organism. Autophagy has been shown to affect aging, which is why it plays such a large role in longevity. The reason for this is twofold. The first reason is that the cells that it acts in are often damaged or injured, and by way of autophagy, the disease or virus that is attempting to infect the organism is unable to spread, allowing the organism to continue living a relatively healthy life. This type of disease control increases the longevity of the organism.

The second reason is that autophagy is essential to maintaining the health of specific tissues and organs, which keeps them running smoothly and functioning at their best, which is also another factor that influences lifespan. If the organs and tissues are healthy, the organism as a whole will be healthy and will keep living.

In these two ways, autophagy plays a large role in the organisms' longevity and lifespan and their cells.

Autophagy can affect the quality of life of a person by maintaining their health and eliminating the disease. Inflammation in the short term helps to get rid of diseases, bacterial infections, and any sort of injury. By effectively eliminating disease and injury on time, the person's quality of life dramatically increases as their health is improved.

When it comes to the quality of life, autophagy has been shown to benefit mental health as well. Intermittent fasting, which induces autophagy, has been shown to decrease instances of depression and food-related disorders such as binge eating. Its benefits for weight loss also have been shown to improve body image, confidence, and overall self-satisfaction in adults who practice it for one month or more.

Other benefits of intermittent fasting include:

- Waistline reduction.

- Enhances psychological function.

- Prevention of neurodegenerative disorders, such as Parkinson's disease, stroke, etc.

- By reducing weight in obese women, intermittent fasting can dial down the symptoms of asthma.

- Tissue damages are reduced during intermittent fasting.

CHAPTER 3. INTERMITTENT FASTING FOR WOMEN OVER 50

According to researchers, intermittent fasting is beneficial for most people who eat during their daytime hours. Prolonged fasting differs from the usual eating style. If someone consumes 3 meals per day, including treats, and they don't work out, they operate on certain

Calories and don't burn their fat reserves at any time. Intermittent fasting allows our bodies to burn the reserved fat storage healthily; nine older women in ten have a form of chronic illness, and nearly eight in ten have more than one chronic disease. So, odds are, eventually, a person will get more. But to live a healthy life, there are measures one should take, and intermittent fasting is one of them.

Many of these chronic illnesses start from being overweight at an older age. The most important aspect of intermittent fasting is its weight loss assistance. Another research found that intermittent fasting induces less muscle loss than the more traditional form of daily restriction of calories. Bear in mind, though, that the primary explanation for its effectiveness is that intermittent fasting allows you to intake fewer calories overall. During your meal times, if you indulge and consume large quantities, you will not lose much weight at all.

Why Start Intermittent Fasting After 50?

Here, excess weight in women can cause these diseases, and intermittent fasting can help counteract them. Furthermore, intermittent fasting can help you control these aspects of living if you are over 50.

Hypertension

With age, blood vessels become less elastic when a person matures. This puts a strain on the mechanism that holds the body's blood. It may indicate why 2 in 3 women over the age of 50 have elevated blood pressure. The best approach to manage hypertension is to lose weight by intermittent fasting.

Diabetes

At least one in 10 women has diabetes. When you grow older, the odds of having the disease increase up. Heart failure, renal disease, blindness, and other complications may arise from diabetes due to excess weight.

Cardiac Condition

A significant source of heart attack is plaque formation in the arteries due to unhealthy eating. It begins in youth, and as one matures, it becomes worse. A large percentage of men and 5.6 percent of women have suffered from heart failure in the 40-58 age range in the U.S. Fasting and eating healthy is a good option to control any cardiovascular diseases.

Obesity

It might be dangerous for the health if one weighs too much for their height; it's not about getting a few extra pounds. More than 20 obesity chronic illnesses are correlated with stroke, asthma, arthritis, cancer, coronary failure, and high blood pressure. At least 30% of the older population is obese.

Arthritis

This condition of the joints was once directly attributed by physicians to the excessive wear and tear of time, and it sure is a cause. Yet biology and lifestyle are likely to have still much to do with it. A lack of physical exercise, diabetes, and becoming overweight may play a role in past joint accidents, too.

Osteoporosis

With old age, bones become weak, especially in women, which may lead to fractures. It impacts nearly 53.9 million Americans over 50 years of age. Some factors that will help: a balanced diet rich in vitamin D and calcium. Lose excess weight by fasting and daily weight-bearing activity, such as walking, jogging, and climbing stairs.

Tumor & Cancers

The greatest risk factor for old age is cancer. The disorder also impacts young adults, but between the ages of 46 and 54, your risk of getting it more than doubles. You can't influence a person's age or genes, but you have a choice in stuff like smoking or living an unhealthy lifestyle. With much of the study focusing on the beneficial impact that fasting has on cancer, fasting over varying periods has often helped older women decrease their risk of severe diseases. The study reported that fasting appears to suppress some cancer-causing pathways and can even delay tumor development.

Menopause

The classic indicators of menopause are hot flashes, insomnia, night sweats, mood swings, and vaginal dryness, burning, and itching. Heart failure and osteoporosis appear to escalate throughout the years of menopause. Often people start prolonged fasting to combat both the long-term and short-term symptoms of menopause. For several post-menopausal women, belly fat, not just for appearance but also for health, is a major concern. The decrease in belly fat resulting from intermittent fasting helped women minimize their likelihood of metabolic syndrome, a series of health conditions that enhance the risk of heart disease and diabetes for a post-menopausal female.

Advantages of Intermittent Fasting for Women Over 50

The benefits of intermittent fasting for women over 50 are limitless; some of them are mentioned here:

Decrease Insulin Resistance

Fasting is one of the most successful strategies to return the insulin receptors to a normal sensitivity level. Understanding the function of insulin plays is one of the biggest keys to learning about fasting and truly understanding every diet. About eating, insulin, the hormone that controls blood sugar, is formed in the pancreas and absorbed into the bloodstream. Insulin allows the body to retain energy as fat until released. Insulin creates fat because the fatter the body stores, the more insulin body makes or vice versa. The cycles during which a person is not eating allow the body time to reduce insulin levels, mainly during intermittent fasting, which changes the fat-storing mechanism. The mechanism goes in reverse, and the body loses weight as insulin levels decrease.

Autophagy is the amazing way cells "eat themselves" to get rid of dead cells and recycle younger parts. Autophagy is often the mechanism by which harmful pathogens, including viruses, bacteria, and other diseases, are killed. As the whole cell is recycled, another step in apoptosis. Your chance of cancer rises without this process when defective cells tend to multiply.

Intermittent Fasting Leads to Detoxification

Many of us have been subjected to contaminants from food and our climate in our lifetime. Many of these containments are processed in our bodies in fat cells. One of the most powerful methods to eliminate contaminants from the body is fasting and eating healthy.

The body's internal clock or Circadian Rhythm of the body controls virtually any mechanism in the body, and a chain of detrimental results will occur when it is disturbed. You adjust the circadian clock of the body while you take a rest from meals.

A Healthy Gut

It is one of the most important aspects of Fasting in that it provides a chance for the digestive tract and intestinal flora to reset. This is critical because the health of the body's digestive system regulates the immune system. There is even more proof that one's moods and emotional wellbeing are co-dependent on the gut microbiota. In recent studies of any area related to health and wellbeing, there has been a lot of hype on how one's gut flora might play an important part. The work of a more powerful immune system is important to a diverse microbiota, and it plays an important role in one's mental wellbeing. It also removes skin problems and reduces cancer danger.

Although the foods you consume have an immense effect on your intestinal health, periodic fasting in the digestive system can be another way to help grow the beneficial bacteria in the gut. Sugar and artificial goods disturb the equilibrium of your digestive tract between the beneficial and detrimental microbiota. Make sure to minimize packaged foods full of refined carbohydrates, sugars, and harmful fats that get the best outcome if you try intermittent fasting. Alternatively, switch to whole grains, plenty of organic vegetables and fruits, and good quality protein.

Intermittent fasting will work better by metabolic switching. Fasting contributes to lower glucose levels in the bloodstream. The body utilizes fat as an energy source instead of sugar after converting the fat into ketones.

Although it's not fasting, several physicians have recorded intermittent fasting advantages by permitting some easy-to-digest foods during the fasting window as fresh fruit. Modifications like this will also provide the essential rest for your metabolic and digestive system.

Losing Weight

It is expected that fasting helps accelerate the loss of excess weight. It also decreases insulin levels such that the body no longer receives the message to store more calories as fat during the state of fasting. Intermittent fasting may contribute to a self-activating decrease in calorie consumption by letting you consume fewer meals. Besides, to promote weight reduction, prolonged fasting affects hormone levels. It enhances noradrenaline or norepinephrine production, which is a fat-burning hormone, lowering insulin and rising growth hormone levels. Intermittent fasting can increase one's metabolic rate due to these changes in hormones. By encouraging one to eat less and activating ketones' production, intermittent fasting induces weight loss by adjusting all calorie calculation factors. In contrast to other weight loss trials, a study showed that this eating method would cause 3-8 percent weight loss in just weeks, which is a substantial percentage. People have lost 4 to 7 percent of their waist circumference; as per the same report, it is helpful for women dealing with menopause and unhealthy stomach fat that builds up over their organs and induces illness.

Other than insulin, during intermittent fasting are two important hormones, leptin and ghrelin. Ghrelin is the hormone of starvation that tells the body when it's hungry. Research shows intermittent fasting can reduce that ghrelin. There is also some evidence suggesting a rise in the leptin hormone, the hormone of satiety. That tells the body when it's full, and there's no more urge to eat.

People would be fuller quicker and hungry less frequently with less ghrelin and more leptin, which may lead to fewer calories eaten and, as a result, weight loss.

Tricks against Hunger Attacks

The best way to curb cravings is intermittent fasting. You don't eat for a certain number of hours each day, typically beginning at 6 am or later in this practice. You can have your main meal at noon and continue eating until 10 pm if you like, but it's generally recommended that you go without eating for 12-16 hours per day.

This practice of eating less often than normal and allowing your body to release stored sugar into your bloodstream is a proven method of curbing cravings and preventing hunger attacks. Intermittent fasting can also help curb the progress of aging, prevent heart disease, reduce cancer risk, and even boost immunity levels.

CHAPTER 4. INTERMITTENT FASTING TYPES

There are countless types of intermittent fasting. There are so many reasons why decide to follow an intermittent fasting lifestyle, and at least as many methods for doing it. Therefore, it is fundamental to set some basic definitions before we go deep in detail.

- Fasting – Giving up the intake of food or anything that has calories for a particular time frame. Normally, some non-caloric beverages and water are allowed.

- Intermittent Fasting – To fast intermittently by adding fasts into your regular meal plan.

- Extended Fasting – Fasting for a drawn-out time. It will, in general, be cultivated for a significant long time.

- Time-Restricted Feeding – Restricting your regular food usage inside a particular time window. This is meant to improve circadian rhythm and general wellness.

Generally, people who do intermittent fasting restrict their eating time and increase their fasting time. To have something like an actual fast, it would need to prop up for over 24 hours since that is the spot most of the benefits start to kick in.

First, let's have an overview of 10 of the main types of intermittent fasting, then we'll go deep into the 6 that better suit women after 50.

24-Hour Fasting

It is the fundamental technique of intermittent fasting—you fast for around 24 hours, and a short time later has a meal. Despite what the name may suggest, you won't actually go through an entire day without eating. Simply eat around the evening, fast all through the next day, and then eat again in the evening.

You can even have your food at the 23-hour check and eat it inside an hour. The idea is to make a very prominent caloric shortage for the day. Most of the benefits will be vain if you, regardless of fasting, binge and put on weight during the eating time frame.

Gradually and occasionally, you can decide to fast according to your physical condition and needs of the moment.

A fit person who works out constantly would require more eating time frames and a few fasting periods.

An overweight person who is sedentary and needs to lose some more weight could follow an intermittent fasting plan as long as they can until they lose the overabundance weight.

16/8 Intermittent Fasting

Martin Berkhan of Lean gains defined 16:8 intermittent fasting. It is used for improving fat loss while not having to go through an extremely demanding process.

You fast for 16 hours and eat your food inside 8. What number of meals you have inside that time length is irrelevant, yet whatever it is recommended to keep them around 2-3.

In my opinion, this should be the base fasting length to concentrate on reliably by everybody. There is no physical need to eat any sooner than that, and the restriction has many benefits.

Many people think it is more straightforward to postpone breakfast by two or three hours and then eat the last meal around early evening. You should not get insane, and it is demanding to observe the fast. The idea is simply to reduce the proportion of time we spend in an eating state and fast for a large portion of the day.

The Warrior Diet

Ori Hofmekler proposes the Warrior Diet. He talks about the benefits of fasting on blood pressure through hormesis.

The warrior diet not only improves your body's physical condition and resistance yet, moreover but also grows your mental attitude and outlook.

The Warrior Diet talks about old warriors like Spartans and Romans who used to remain on an empty stomach all through the day and eat in the evening. During daylight, they used to stroll around with 40 pounds of armor, build fortresses, and bear the hot sun of the Mediterranean, while having just a quick bite. They would have a huge supper around evening time consisting of stews, meat, bread, and many other things.

In the Warrior Diet, you fast for around 20 hours, have a short high power workout, and eat your food during a 4 hours window. Overall, it would merge either two minor meals with a break or one single huge supper.

One Meal a Day OMAD

One Meal a Day Diet, also called OMAD, simply consists of eating just one big meal every day

With OMAD, you regularly fast around 21-23 hours and eat your food inside a 1-2 hour time slot. This is remarkable for dieting since you can feel full and satisfied once the eating time comes.

It is unmatched for losing fat; be that as it may, not ideal for muscle improvement because of time for protein production and anabolism.

36-Hour Fasting

In the past, people would quite commonly go a couple of days without eating; they probably suffered and yet even thrived. Today, the average person can't bear to skip breakfast or go to bed hungry.

For over 24 hours is the spot where all the magic begins; the more you stay in a fasted state and experience hardship, the more your body is forced to trigger its supply systems that start to draw on fat stores, bolster rejuvenating microorganisms, and reuse old wrecked cell material through the system of autophagy.

It takes, at any rate, an entire day to see significant signs of autophagy. Yet, you can speed it up by eating low carb before starting the fast, rehearsing on an unfilled stomach, and drinking some homemade teas that facilitate the challenge.

For 36 hours, it's not really that annoying. You fundamentally eat the night before, don't eat anything during the day, go to sleep on an empty stomach, then wake up the next day, fast a few more hours, and begin eating again.

To make the fasting more straightforward, there are mineral water, plain coffee, green tea, and some homemade teas.

48-Hour Fasting

In case you made it to the 36-hour mark, why not give it a try to fast for a straight 48 hours.

It is only annoying getting through the change of habits. Once you overcome this obstacle, which generally occurs around your usual dinnertime, it gets a lot more straightforward.

The moment your body goes into an increasingly significant ketosis phase and autophagy starts, you will overcome hunger, feel very mentally clear, and have greater mindfulness and focus.

The most problematic bit of any complete fast is around the 24-hour mark. If you can make it to fall asleep and wake up the next day, you have set yourself prepared for fasting for a significant time with no issues from that moment onward. You essentially need to get over this hidden obstacle.

Going to bed hungry sounds disturbing; in any case, this is what a huge part of the world's population does daily. This could make you think about your own luck and feel thankful for having food anytime you want.

Expanded Fasting (3-7 Days)

48-hours fasting would give you a short ride in autophagy and some fat consumption. To genuinely get the deep health benefits of fasting, you would have to fast for three or more days.

It has been shown that 72-hours of fasting can reset the immune system in mice. However, studies on humans have not confirmed that conclusion; also, there may be some issues in prolonged fasting that are not under severe medical control.

Three to five days is the perfect time frame for autophagy, after which you may begin to see unwanted losses in bulk and muscle. Fasting for seven or more days is not generally suggested. Most people do not need to fast any longer than that since it may make them lose muscle tissue.

Fit people may want to focus on three-four of these expanded fasts every year, to propel cell recovery and clean out the body. Notwithstanding a healthy eating routine without any junk food, I do it anyway four times a year because of their tremendous benefits.

In case you are overweight or experience the negative effects of some illness, then longer fasts can really help you get back in health. Fast for three to five days, have a little refreshment break and repeat the plan until needed. I'll never say that enough; if you decide to go through this kind of longer fasting, be always sure of what you are doing and consult a doctor for any doubt.

Alternate Day Fasting

Alternate Day Fasting, as for the 5:2 Diet, is a very common type of fasting. Are they fully considered fasting, despite allowing the intake of 500/660 calories a day on fasting days? Well, yes, they are, since these limited amounts of calories are only intended to help extend perseverance.

To have a sporadic caloric intake will not enable the whole of the physiological benefits of fasting to fully manifest. It would limit a part of the effect. In any case, a strict limitation is important for both your physiology and mind.

Everybody can fast. It is just that someone cannot psychologically bear the weight of not eating. Fasting mimicking diets and alternate-day fasting in this respect.

Fasting Mimicking Diet (FMD)

The Fasting Mimicking Diet can be used every so often. Commonly, people who cannot actually fast, like old people or some recovering patients follow it.

Fasting mimicking diet has been shown to reduce blood pressure, lower insulin, and cover IGF-1, all of which have positive life length benefits. Regardless, these effects are likely an immediate consequence of the huge caloric restriction.

During the Fasting Mimicking Diet, you would eat low protein, moderate carb, and moderate fat foods like mushroom soup, olives, kale wafers, and some nut bars. The idea is to give you something to eat while keeping the calories as low as reasonable. In most cases, again, this is more about satisfying people's psychological needs of eating than the physical ones.

With zero calories would be just as effective, and it would keep up more muscle tissue by increasingly significant ketosis. To thwart the unwanted loss of lean mass, you can adapt the macronutrient taken in during Fasting Mimicking Diet and make them more ketogenic by cutting down the carbs and increasing the fats.

Protein Sparing Modified Fasting

Protein-Sparing Modified Fast (PSMF) is a low carb, low fat, high protein type of diet that helps to get increasingly fit quite fast while keeping muscle toned.

Lean mass is a significant matter of stress for healthy people, especially in case they are endeavoring to do intermittent fasting.

A catabolic stressor will, over the long term, lead to muscle loss; notwithstanding, the loss rate is a lot lower than people may imagine. To prevent that from happening, you have to stay in ketosis and lower the body's appetite for glucose.

PSMF is absolutely going to keep up more muscle than the fasting-mimicking diet. Yet, there's the danger of staying out of ketosis in case you are already eating many proteins preparing yourself for muscle catabolism.

CHAPTER 5. BREAKFASTS

1. <u>Turmeric Chicken and Kale Salad with Food, Lemon and Honey</u>

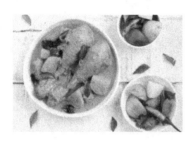

Preparation Time: 20 minutes

Cooking Time: 15 minutes

Servings: 4

Ingredients:

<u>For the chicken:</u>

- 1 teaspoon of clarified butter or 1 tablespoon of coconut oil

- ½ medium brown onion, diced

- 250-300 g / 9 ounces of minced chicken meat or diced chicken legs

- 1 large garlic clove, diced

- 1 teaspoon of turmeric powder

- 1 teaspoon of lime zest

- ½ lime juice

- ½ teaspoon of salt + pepper

For the salad:

- 6 stalks of broccoli or 2 cups of broccoli flowers

- 2 tablespoons of pumpkin seeds (seeds)

- 3 large cabbage leaves, stems removed and chopped

- ½ sliced avocado

- Handful of fresh coriander leaves, chopped

- Handful of fresh parsley leaves, chopped

For the dressing:

- 3 tablespoons of lime juice

- 1 small garlic clove, diced or grated

- 3 tablespoons of virgin olive oil (I used 1 tablespoon of avocado oil and 2 tablespoons of EVO)

- 1 teaspoon of raw honey

- ½ teaspoon of whole or Dijon mustard

- ½ teaspoon of sea salt with pepper

Directions:

1. Heat the coconut oil in a pan. Add the onion and sauté over medium heat for 4-5 minutes, until golden brown. Add the minced chicken and garlic and stir 2-3 minutes over medium-high heat, separating.

2. Add your turmeric, lime zest, lime juice, salt, and pepper, and cook, stirring consistently, for another 3-4 minutes. Set the ground beef aside.

3. While your chicken is cooking, put a small saucepan of water to the boil. Add your broccoli and cook for 2 minutes. Rinse with cold water and cut into 3-4 pieces each.

4. Add the pumpkin seeds to the chicken pan and toast over medium heat for 2 minutes, frequently stirring to avoid burning. Season with a little salt. Set aside. Raw pumpkin seeds are also good to use.

5. Put the chopped cabbage in a salad bowl and pour it over the dressing. Using your hands, mix, and massage the cabbage with the dressing. This will soften the cabbage, a bit like citrus juice with fish or beef Carpaccio: it "cooks" it a little.

6. Finally, mix the cooked chicken, broccoli, fresh herbs, pumpkin seeds, and avocado slices.

Nutrition:

- Calories 232 kcal Fat 11 g Fiber 9 g Carbs 8 g

- Protein 14 g

2. <u>Buckwheat Spaghetti with Chicken Cabbage in Miso Sauce</u>

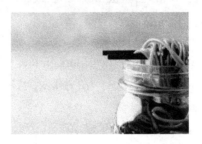

Preparation Time: 15 minutes

Cooking Time: 15 minutes

Servings: 2

Ingredients:

<u>For the noodles:</u>

- 2-3 handfuls of cabbage leaves (removed from the stem and cut)

- Buckwheat noodles 150g / 5oz (100% buckwheat, without wheat)

- 3-4 shiitake mushrooms, sliced

- 1 teaspoon of coconut oil or butter

- 1 brown onion, finely chopped

- 1 medium chicken breast, sliced or diced

- 1 long red pepper, thinly sliced (seeds in or out depending on how hot you like it)

- 2 large garlic cloves, diced

- 2-3 tablespoons of Tamari sauce (gluten-free soy sauce)

- Sea salt

For the miso dressing:

- 1 tablespoon and a half of fresh organic miso

- 1 tablespoon of Tamari sauce

- 1 tablespoon of extra virgin olive oil

- 1 teaspoon of sesame oil (optional)

Directions:

1. Boil a medium saucepan of water. Add the cabbage and cook for 1 minute, until it is wilted. Remove and reserve, but reserve the water and return to boiling. Add your Buckwheat noodles and cook according to the directions on the package (usually about 5 minutes). Rinse with cold water and reserve.

2. In the meantime, fry the shiitake mushrooms in a little butter or coconut oil (about a teaspoon) for 2-3 minutes, until its color is lightly browned on each side. Sprinkle with sea salt and reserve.

3. In that same pan, heat more coconut oil or lard over medium-high heat. Fry the onion and the red pepper for 2-3 minutes, and

then add the chicken pieces. Cook for 5 minutes on medium heat, stirring a few times, then add the garlic, tamari sauce, and a little water. Cook for another 2-3 minutes, stirring continuously until your chicken is cooked.

4. Finally, add the cabbage and Buckwheat noodles and stir the chicken to warm it.

5. Stir the miso sauce and sprinkle the noodles at the end of the cooking, in this way you will keep alive all the beneficial probiotics in the miso.

Nutrition:

- Calories 305 kcal

- Fat 11 g

- Fiber 7 g

- Carbs 9 g

- Protein 12 g

3. <u>Sheet Pan Eggs with Veggies and Parmesan</u>

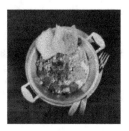

Preparation Time: 5 minutes

Cooking Time: 15 minutes

Servings: 4

Ingredients:

- 6 large eggs, whisked

- Salt and pepper small red pepper, diced

- 1 small yellow onion, chopped

- 1/2 cup of diced mushrooms

- 1/2 cup of diced zucchini

- 1/2 cup of freshly grated parmesan cheese

Directions:

1. Now, preheat the oven to 350 ° F and grease cooking spray on a rimmed baking sheet.

2. In a cup, whisk the eggs with salt and pepper until sparkling.

3. In a bowl put the peppers, onions, mushrooms, and the zucchinis until well mixed.

4. Pour the mixture into a baking sheet and scatter over a layer of evenness.

5. Sprinkle with parmesan, and bake until the egg is set for 13 to 16 minutes.

6. Let it cool down slightly, then cut to squares for serving.

Nutrition:

- Calories 180 kcal

- Fat 10 g

- Protein 14.5 g

- Carbohydrates 5 g

- Fiber 1 g

- Net Carbs 4 g

4. <u>Almond Butter Muffins</u>

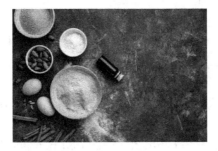

Preparation Time: 10 minutes

Cooking Time: 25 minutes

Servings: 6

Ingredients:

- 1 cup of almond flour

- 1/2 cup of powdered Erythritol

- 2 teaspoons of baking powder

- 1/4 teaspoon of salt

- 3/4 cup of almond butter, warmed

- 3/4 cup of unsweetened almond milk 3 large eggs

Directions:

1. Now, preheat the oven to 350 ° F, and line a paper liner muffin pan.

2. In a mixing bowl, whisk the almond flour and the Erythritol, baking powder, and salt.

3. Whisk the almond milk, almond butter, and eggs together in a separate bowl.

4. Drop the wet ingredients into the dry until just mixed together.

5. Spoon the batter into the prepared pan and bake for 22 to 25 minutes until clean comes out the knife inserted in the middle.

6. Cook the muffins in the pan for 5 minutes. Then, switch onto a cooling rack with wire.

Nutrition:

- Calories 135 kcal

- Fat 11 g

- Protein 6 g

- Carbohydrates 4 g

- Fiber 2 g

- Net Carbs 2 g

5. <u>Sheet Pan Eggs with Ham and Pepper Jack</u>

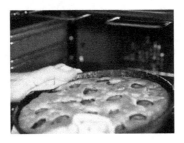

Preparation Time: 5 minutes

Cooking Time: 15 minutes

Servings: 6

Ingredients:

- 12 large eggs, whisked

- Salt and pepper

- 2 cups of diced ham

- 1 cup of shredded pepper jack cheese

Directions:

1. Now, preheat the oven to 350 °F and grease a rimmed baking sheet w/ cooking spray.

2. Whisk the eggs in a mixing bowl then add salt and pepper until frothy.

3. Stir in the ham and cheese and mix until well combined.

4. Pour the mixture into baking sheets and spread it into an even layer.

5. Bake for 12 to 15 mins until the egg is set.

6. Let cool slightly then cut it into squares to serve.

Nutrition:

- Calories 235 kcal

- Fat 15 g

- Protein 21 g

- Carbs 2.5 g

- Fiber 0.5 g

- Net Carbs 2g

6. <u>Counterfeit Bagels</u>

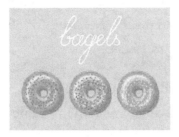

Preparation Time: 15 minutes

Cooking Time: 17 minutes

Servings: 10

Ingredients:

- 1½ cups of blanched almond flour

- 1 tablespoon of baking powder

- 2½ cups of shredded whole milk mozzarella cheese

- 3 ounces of full-fat cream cheese, softened

- 4 large eggs, whisked 2 tablespoons of Everything but the Bagel seasoning

- 1 tablespoon of unsalted butter, melted

Directions:

1. Preheat oven to 400 °F. Line a baking sheet with parchment paper. In a bowl, mix almond flour and baking powder.

2. In a medium microwave-safe bowl, mix mozzarella cheese, cream cheese, and whisked eggs. Microwave cheese mixture 1 minute. Stir and microwave again for 30 seconds. Let mixture cool until okay to handle.

3. Combine dry ingredients into a cheese mixture. Work quickly, stirring with a sturdy spatula or bamboo spoon to create a dough. Shape dough into approximately ¾"-thick snakes, and then form into ten bagels.

4. Place bagels on a prepared baking sheet and sprinkle tops with seasoning. Bake 15 minutes until browning on top. Remove bagels from the oven, brush with melted butter, and serve.

Nutrition:

- Calories 236 kcal

- Fat 18 g

- Protein 11 g

7. Starbucks Egg Bites

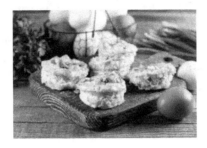

Preparation Time: 5 minutes

Cooking Time: 30 minutes

Servings: 6

Ingredients:

- 5 large eggs, whisked

- 1 cup of shredded Swiss cheese

- 1 cup of full-fat cottage cheese

- 1/8 teaspoon of salt

- 1/8 teaspoon of black pepper

- strips no-sugar-added bacon, cooked and crumbled

Directions:

1. Prepare the oven to 350 °F. In a big bowl, scourge eggs, Swiss cheese, cottage cheese, salt, and pepper. Portion six equal

amounts of mixture into well-greased muffin tins (or use cupcake liners).

2. Sprinkle with bacon bits. Bake 30 minutes until eggs are completely cooked. Take out Starbucks Egg Bites from the oven and serve warm.

Nutrition:

- Calories 182 kcal

- Fat 11 g

- Protein 16 g

8. <u>DLK Bulletproof Coffee</u>

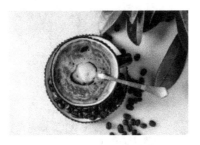

Preparation Time: 2 minutes

Cooking Time: 0 minutes

Servings: 1

Ingredients:

- 1 tablespoon MCT oil

- 8 ounces hot brewed coffee

Directions:

1. Add MCT oil to coffee and blend using a hand immersion blender until the froth whips up. This will help prevent the dreaded MCT oil "lip gloss."

2. Serve.

Nutrition:

- Calories 132 kcal

- Fat 14g Protein 0g

9. <u>Green Monster Smoothie</u>

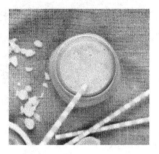

Preparation Time: 3 minutes

Cooking Time: 0 minute

Servings: 1

Ingredients:

- 1 cup of ice 1 cup of chopped fresh spinach

- ½ cup of fresh raspberries (1-gram) packets of 0g net carb sweetener 1 cup of unsweetened almond milk

Directions:

1. Throw all the ingredients in a food processor for 30–60 seconds until ice is blended.

Nutrition:

- Calories 67 kcal

- Fat 3 g Protein 3 g

10. <u>Radish Hash Brown</u>

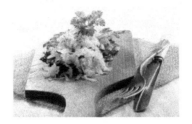

Preparation Time: 10 minutes

Cooking Time: 40 minutes

Servings: 10

Ingredients:

- 2 pounds of radishes, trimmed

- 4 tablespoons of radishes

- olive oil 2 large egg, whisked

- 1/8 teaspoon of salt 1/8 teaspoon of black pepper

Directions:

1. Shred radish using a food processor or hand grater and squeeze out extra moisture using cheesecloth or clean dishtowel. In a medium skillet over medium heat, heat oil. Add radishes and stir often. Sauté 20–30 minutes until golden. Take away from heat and place into a medium bowl.

2. Stir whisked egg into a bowl with salt and pepper. Form ten small pancakes. Add back to hot skillet. Heat 3–5 minutes on each side until solid and brown. Serve warm.

Nutrition:

- Calories 63 kcal

- Fat 6 g

- Protein 1 g

11. <u>Cloud Bread</u>

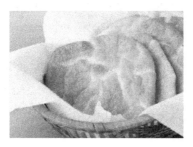

Preparation Time: 10 minutes

Cooking Time: 36 minutes

Servings: 6

Ingredients:

- 3 tablespoons of full-fat cream cheese, softened

- 3 large eggs

- 1 tablespoon of 0g net carb sweetener

- ¼ teaspoon of baking powder

Directions:

1. Preheat oven to 300 °F. Line a baking sheet with parchment paper. In a medium microwave-safe bowl, heat up cream cheese for 30 seconds. Stir and microwave again for 15 seconds.

2. Crack eggs and separate into two different medium bowls. Add cream cheese to the bowl containing the yolks, and add 0g net carb sweetener to the egg whites. Combine baking powder with

egg whites and beat with an electric mixer until stiff peaks form, about 3–4 minutes at high speed. Make sure there is no yolk in the bowl, as it will not mix properly.

3. Blend egg yolk mixture with a whisk or hand mixer until well blended and smooth. Cream cheese must be completely mixed in. Gently fold egg yolk mixture into egg white mixture until fully combined.

4. Spoon mixture into six even patties on a baking sheet. Bake 30–35 minutes until tops are golden. Let cool for 10 minutes and lift off the parchment paper (easiest to do when rolls are still warm). Serve.

Nutrition:

- Calories 60 kcal

- Fat 4 g

- Protein 4 g

12. OG Breadsticks

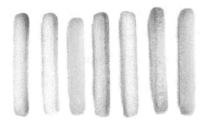

Preparation Time: 15 minutes

Cooking Time: 24 minutes

Servings: 4

Ingredients:

- 4 cups of riced cauliflower

- 2 cups of shredded whole milk mozzarella cheese,

- 2 large eggs, whisked

- 1 tablespoon of garlic powder

- 1 tablespoon of Italian seasoning

Directions:

1. Preheat oven to 450 °F. Line a baking sheet with parchment paper. In a medium microwave-safe bowl, microwave the cauliflower for 3–4 minutes to soften. Put in a colander and let cool 5 minutes.

2. Toss the cauliflower into a food processor and pulse until the consistency becomes a gritty pulp. Remove excess water by squeezing in a cheesecloth. Pour cauliflower into a medium mixing bowl and add the rest of the ingredients, leaving out ¼ cup of cheese to add at the end. Thoroughly mix the ingredients in the bowl until they form a big ball of dough.

3. Place dough on a baking sheet and top with another sheet of parchment paper. Roll out dough until it's about ¼" thick. The shape doesn't matter. Don't worry if it's a little watery; the oven will firm it up.

4. Take off the top part of parchment paper and bake for 20 minutes until it shows signs of browning. Remove and top with remaining cheese. Cut with a pizza cutter and serve warm.

Nutrition:

- Calories 231 kcal

- Fat 14 g

- Protein 18 g

13. <u>Fettuccini Alfredo</u>

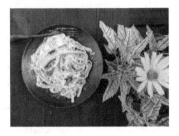

Preparation Time: 50 minutes

Cooking Time: 28 minutes

Servings: 8

Ingredients:

- Keto Noodles

- 3 cups of fine unblanched almond flour

- 1/3 cup of coconut flour 6 teaspoons of xanthan gum

- 6 teaspoons of apple cider vinegar

- 3 large eggs, whisked 1 tablespoon of water, if needed for consistency Alfredo Sauce

- ½ cup of unsalted butter cloves garlic, peeled and minced

- 2 ounces full-fat cream cheese, softened

- 1½ cups of heavy whipping cream

- 1½ cups of grated Parmesan cheese

- ¼ teaspoon of salt

Directions:

1. Preheat oven to 375 °F. Line a baking sheet with parchment paper. In a large mixing bowl, mix dry noodle ingredients together. Add vinegar and eggs and mix thoroughly. If the dough is too thick, add a bit of water (very slowly) to reach desired consistency.

2. Refrigerate dough for 30 minutes. Put the chilled dough ball in the center of the baking sheet and cover the dough with a second piece of parchment paper. Using a rolling pin, roll to desired noodle thickness.

3. Remove the top piece of parchment paper. With a pizza cutter, cut dough into thin strips for noodles. Bake 20 minutes until noodles are firm, but loose, like pasta.

4. Make the sauce: Melt butter in a medium saucepan over medium heat. Add garlic and cook 3 minutes until soft. Add remaining sauce ingredients while stirring until cheese is completely melted and a thick, uniform sauce forms (about 5 minutes).

5. Top each Keto noodle serving with ½ cup Alfredo sauce. Serve.

Nutrition:

- Calories 701 kcal

- Fat 60 g Protein 20 g

14.   <u>Coated Cauliflower Head</u>

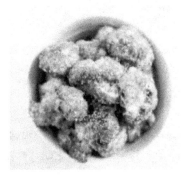

Preparation Time: 10 minutes

Cooking Time: 40 minutes

Servings: 6

Ingredients:

- 2-pound of cauliflower head

- 3 tablespoons of olive oil

- 1 tablespoon of butter, softened

- 1 teaspoon of ground coriander

- 1 teaspoon of salt

- 1 egg, whisked

- 1 teaspoon of dried cilantro

- 1 teaspoon of dried oregano

- 1 teaspoon of tahini paste

Directions:

1. Trim the cauliflower head if needed.

2. Preheat oven to 350F.

3. In the mixing bowl, mix up together olive oil, softened butter, ground coriander, salt, whisked egg, dried cilantro, dried oregano, and tahini paste.

4. Then brush the cauliflower head with this mixture generously and transfer it in the tray.

5. Bake the cauliflower head for 40 minutes.

6. Brush it with the remaining oil mixture every 10 minutes.

Nutrition:

- Calories 131 kcal

- Fat 10.3 g

- Fiber 4 g

- Carbs 8.4 g

- Protein 4.1 g

15. <u>Spinach with Baked Eggs</u>

Preparation Time: 5 minutes

Cooking Time: 15 minutes

Servings: 2

Ingredients:

- 2 teaspoons of Olive oil

- 10 cups of Spinach

- 2 teaspoons of Garlic

- 1 cup of Cheese, shredded

- 2 Eggs

Directions:

1. Preheat the oven to 325 °F.

2. In a skillet heat oil, add 1 tsp. of garlic, spinach, and sauté for 3-4 minutes.

3. Add ¼-cup of cheese and divide mixture into 2 ramekins.

4. Crack one egg over each spinach mixture.

5. Bake for 12-15 minutes.

6. Add salt, pepper, and serve.

Nutrition:

- Calories: 205.7 kcal

- Fat 13.5 g

- Carbs: 3.6 g

- Protein: 17.5 g

16. Purple Eggplant Lasagna

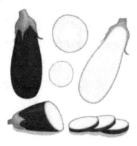

Preparation Time: 30 minutes

Cooking Time: 68 minutes

Servings: 10

Ingredients:

- 1-pound of lean ground beef

- ½ medium onion, peeled and chopped

- ¼ cup of dried parsley 1 cup of no-sugar-added pasta sauce

- 1-pound of whole milk ricotta cheese

- 1 large egg 1/8 teaspoon of salt

- 1/8 teaspoon of black pepper 1 large eggplant

- 3 cups of whole milk mozzarella cheese

Directions:

1. Preheat oven to 350 °F. Grease a 13" × 9" casserole dish.

2. In a big skillet, cook beef for 10–15 minutes over medium heat. Drain excess fat. Stir in onion and parsley and cook 2–3 minutes until soft. Mix in the pasta sauce and bring to boil while stirring frequently (3–5 minutes). Turn off heat.

3. In a medium bowl, blend ricotta cheese and egg then season with salt and pepper. Cut unpeeled eggplant lengthwise in thin slices no more than 1/8-inch. This would be enough to complete 2 layers in your baking dish.

4. In the casserole dish, add ¼" layer of ricotta cheese mixture to avoid eggplant from sticking. On top of ricotta layer, create an even layer of half the eggplant slices.

5. Arrange a layer of half of the remaining ricotta cheese mixture. Next, spread 1 cup of mozzarella cheese, then half of the meat/pasta sauce and the remaining eggplant, following the rest of the ricotta mixture and leftover meat mixture. Sprinkle with the remaining 1-cup of mozzarella cheese.

6. Cover the dish with aluminum foil. Bake 40 minutes. Take off the foil and cook an additional 5 minutes to brown cheese. Let cool 15 minutes, then cut and serve.

Nutrition:

- Calories 250 kcal

- Fat 14 g Protein 21 g

17.   Summer Swiss Chard

Preparation Time: 5 minutes

Cooking Time: 15 minutes

Servings: 4

Ingredients:

- 1 pound of Swiss chard

- 3 tablespoons of Olive oil

- 1 cup of Onion, diced

- Salt

- ½ teaspoon of Oregano

- 3 tablespoons of Red-wine vinegar

- Salt

- Pepper

Directions:

1. Chop the chard and set it aside.

2. Heat the olive oil in a skillet over medium heat.

3. Add the diced onion, a pinch of salt, and oregano and cook until the onions are tender.

4. Add the chopped chard and sauté for a few minutes and then remove from heat.

5. Stir in the vinegar and season with salt and pepper.

Nutrition:

- Calories 132 kcal

- Fat 11 g

- Protein 3 g

- Carbs 8 g

18.   Strawberry-banana Smoothie

Preparation Time: 3 minutes

Cooking Time: 2 minutes

Servings: 2

Ingredients:

- 1 Banana

- 1 cup of Strawberries, frozen and sliced

- 1 cup of vanilla yogurt, frozen

- ¼ cup of orange juice

- 1 teaspoon of Honey

Directions:

1. Place all the ingredients in a blender and blend until smooth.

2. Pour into two glasses and serve as a quick breakfast.

Nutrition:

- Calories 248 kcal Fat 4g Protein 4 g

- Carbs 50 g

19. Pizza Hut Cheesy Breadsticks

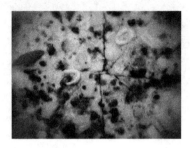

Preparation Time: 15 minutes

Cooking Time: 14 minutes

Servings: 12

Ingredients:

- 2 cups of shredded whole milk mozzarella, divided

- 1 ounce of full-fat cream cheese, softened

- ½ cup of blanched almond flour

- 3 tablespoons of coconut flour

- 1 large egg, whisked 1/3 cup of grated Parmesan cheese

- 1 teaspoon of dried parsley

Directions:

1. Preheat oven to 425 °F. In a large microwave-safe bowl, place 1½ cups mozzarella and cream cheese. Heat in microwave for 1½ minutes, stirring every 30 seconds.

2. Add almond flour, coconut flour, and egg. Fold until blended. Let the dough cool for handling. Create dough into a ball and arrange it between two sheets of parchment paper. Roll out to approximately ¼" thick. Peel the top layer of paper and put the dough, while still on the bottom piece of parchment paper, on a baking sheet. Sprinkle ¼-cup of mozzarella over dough. Bake 5–7 minutes until the edges of the dough are golden. Take the dough out of the oven. Sprinkle with remaining mozzarella and Parmesan cheese. Bake 5 minutes until cheese is melted.

3. Remove from oven and garnish with parsley. Cut into twelve equal breadsticks using a pizza cutter. Serve warm.

Nutrition:

- Calories 115 kcal

- Fat 7 g

- Protein 7 g

CHAPTER 6. LUNCH

20. Basil Mozzarella Eggs

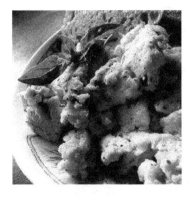

Preparation Time: 5 minutes

Cooking Time: 20 minutes **Servings:** 4

Ingredients:

- 2 tablespoons of butter, melted

- 6 teaspoons of basil pesto

- 1 cup of mozzarella cheese, grated

- 6 eggs, whisked 2 tablespoons of basil, chopped

- A pinch of salt and black pepper

Directions:

1. In a bowl, put and combine all the ingredients except the butter and whisk them well.

2. Preheat your Air Fryer at 360 ° F, drizzle the butter on the bottom, spread the eggs mix, cook for 20 minutes, and serve for breakfast.

Nutrition:

- Calories 207 kcal

- Fat 14 g

- Fiber 3 g

- Carbohydrates 4 g

- Protein 8 g

21. <u>Spinach-Mandarin Salad</u>

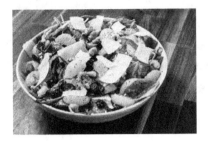

Preparation Time: 20 minutes

Cooking Time: 0 minutes **Servings:** 8

Ingredients:

- 2 cups of fresh spinach

- ½ cup of dried sweetened cranberries

- 5-ounces of drained water chestnuts, drained

- 1 cup of mandarin oranges, drained

- 1 medium-sized apple, cut into wedges

- ¼ cup of crunchy chow Mein noodles

- 1 teaspoon of black pepper ¼ cup of vinaigrette salad dressing

Directions:

1. Using a 1-quart serving bowl, place in the washed and drained spinach, then spread on top the dried cranberries. Add the water

chestnuts, apple wedges, chow Mein noodles, and mandarin oranges.

2. Sprinkle pepper over the top, then cover and store in the refrigerator to chill. Use ¼-cup of vinaigrette salad dressing to toss over the mixture lightly, and then serve.

Nutrition:

- Calories 157 kcal

- Protein 2 g

- Carbohydrates 31 g

- Fat 4 g

- Sodium 145 mg

- Potassium 232 mg

- Phosphorus 32 mg

22. <u>Wholesome Keto Avo-Burgers</u>

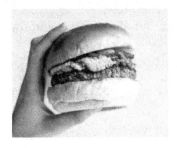

Preparation Time: 5 minutes

Cooking Time: 5 minutes

Servings: 2

Ingredients:

- 2 avocados

- 2 eggs

- 2 tablespoons of chopped lettuce

- 2 tablespoons of mayonnaise

- 4 strips of bacon

Directions:

1. Bring out a skillet pan, put it over medium heat and when hot, add bacon strips and cook for 5 minutes until crispy.

2. Put bacon to a plate lined with paper towels, crack an egg into the pan, and cook for at least 2 to 4 minutes, until fried to the desired level; fry the remaining egg in the same manner.

3. Prepare sandwiches and for this, cut each avocado in half widthwise, remove the pit, and scoop out the flesh.

4. Fill the hollow of two avocado halves with mayonnaise, then top each half with 1 tablespoon of chopped lettuce, 2 bacon strips, and a fried egg, and then cover with the second half of avocado.

5. Sprinkle sesame seeds on avocados and serve.

Nutrition:

- Calories 205 kcal

- Fats 19 g

- Protein 8 g

- Carbohydrates 1 g

23. <u>Cheesy Brussels sprouts and Eggs</u>

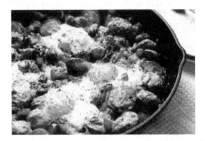

Preparation Time: 5 minutes

Cooking Time: 20 minutes

Servings: 4

Ingredients:

- 1 tablespoon of olive oil

- 1 pound of Brussels sprouts, shredded

- 4 eggs, whisked

- ½-cup of coconut cream

- Salt and black pepper to the taste

- 1 tablespoon of chives, chopped

- ¼ cup of cheddar cheese, shredded

Directions:

1. Preheat the Air Fryer at 360 °F and grease it with the oil.

2. Spread the Brussels sprouts on the bottom of the fryer, then add the eggs mixed with the rest of the ingredients, toss a bit, and cook for 20 minutes.

3. Divide between plates and serve.

Nutrition:

- Calories 242 kcal

- Fat 12 g

- Fiber 3 g

- Carbohydrates 5 g

- Protein 9 g

24. <u>Eggs in Pepper</u>

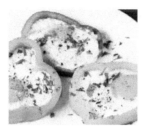

Preparation Time: 20 minutes

Cooking Time: 6 minutes

Servings: 2

Ingredients:

- 6 eggs

- 1 bell pepper, sliced into ¼ in. rings

- Salt and ground black pepper, to taste

- 2 tablespoons of chopped chives and parsley

- 2 tablespoons of olive oil

Directions:

1. Heat a frying pan to medium heat temperature and grease it lightly.

2. Place bell pepper rings in the pan for 2 minutes.

3. Flip the rings and crack an egg in the middle of the rings.

4. Add salt and pepper.

5. Cook 2-4 minutes.

6. Repeat with other pepper rings and eggs.

7. Garnish with parsley and chives.

Nutrition:

- Calories 157 kcal

- Total Fats 12 g

- Net Carbs 6 g

- Protein 12 g

- Fiber 6.3 g

25.   Naan Bread and Butter

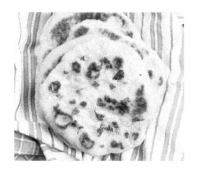

Preparation Time: 20 minutes

Cooking Time: 5 minutes

Servings: 2

Ingredients:

- 7 tablespoons of coconut oil

- ¾ cup of coconut flour

- 2 tablespoons of psyllium powder

- ½ teaspoon of baking powder

- Salt, to taste

- 2 cups of hot water

- Some coconut oil, for frying

- 2 garlic cloves, peeled and minced

- 5 ounces of butter

Directions:

1. In a bowl, combine the coconut flour with baking powder, salt, and psyllium powder, and stir.

2. Add the coconut oil and the hot water and knead the dough. Set aside for 5 minutes, divide into 6 balls, and flatten them on a working surface.

3. In a pan, pour coconut oil the heat it over medium-high heat, add the naan bread to the pan, fry it until golden brown then transfer them to a plate.

4. Heat up a pan with the butter over medium-high heat, add the garlic, salt, and pepper, stir, and cook for 2 minutes.

5. Brush the naan bread with this mixture, pour the rest into a bowl, and serve.

Nutrition:

- Calories 140 kcal

- Total Fats 9 g

- Net Carbs 3 g

- Protein 4 g

- Fiber 1 g

26. <u>Tuna Salad</u>

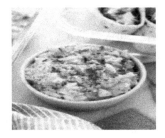

Preparation Time: 10 minutes

Cooking Time: 4 minutes

Servings: 2

Ingredients:

- 2 tablespoons of sour cream

- 12 ounces of canned tuna in olive oil

- 4 leeks, diced

- A pinch of red chili flakes

- 1 tablespoon of capers

- 8 tablespoons of mayonnaise

- Salt and ground black pepper, to taste

Directions:

1. Mix all the ingredients listed in one salad bowl.

2. Stir well and serve.

Nutrition:

- Calories 160 kcal

- Total Fats 3 g

- Net Carbs 2 g

- Protein 6 g

- Fiber 1 g

27.   Low-Carb Muffins with Whey Protein

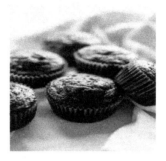

Preparation Time: 10 minutes

Cooking Time: 30 minutes

Servings: 6

Ingredients:

- 1 egg

- 4 teaspoons of Whey Protein (Chocolate)

- 4 tablespoons of low-fat milk

- 1 teaspoon of cacao

- ½ teaspoon of vanilla sugar

- ½ pack of baking powder

Directions:

1. In one bowl, whisk 1 egg with milk and vanilla sugar. Combine them well.

2. Gradually, add whey, cacao, and baking powder to the mixture. Mix constantly.

3. Pour the resulting mixture into muffin molds.

4. Bake at 220°F for 30 minutes. Enjoy!

Nutrition:

- Calories 112 kcal

- Total Fats 5 g

- Net Carbs 6 g

- Protein 1.2 g

- Fiber 3.3 g

28. <u>Spinach Rolls</u>

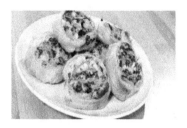

Preparation Time: 10 minutes

Cooking Time: 10 minutes

Servings: 6

Ingredients:

- 7 ounces of white meat, cut into small cubes

- 1 cup of spinach

- 4 eggs

- 7 ounces of cream cheese

- ½ teaspoon of sodium bicarbonate

- 4 tablespoons of flour

Directions:

1. Cook spinach and meat in water (Separately).

2. Whisk 3 eggs with 4 tablespoons of flour, sodium, salt, and 2 tablespoons of cheese, and ½ cup of cooked spinach.

3. Mix them well and bake at 250 °F for 10 minutes.

4. Meanwhile, dissolve a pinch of salt in water. Add ½ cup of cooked spinach, meat, and 1 egg. Cook the mixture in a cooking pot until the meat is done.

5. Cut baked dough into smaller sizes, fill them with the cooked mixture, and roll. Enjoy!

Nutrition:

- Calories 123 kcal

- Total Fats 4 g

- Net Carbs 8 g

- Protein 3 g

- Fiber 2.4 g

29. <u>Pesto Scramble</u>

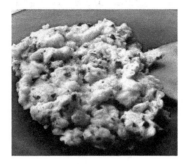

Preparation Time: 5 minutes

Cooking Time: 5 minutes

Servings: 2

Ingredients:

- 1 tablespoon of basil pesto

- 1 tablespoon of unsalted butter

- 1/8 teaspoon of ground black pepper

- 1/8 teaspoon of salt

- 2 eggs

- 2 tablespoons of grated cheddar cheese

Directions:

1. Crack eggs in a bowl, add cheese, black pepper, salt, and pesto, and whisk until combined.

2. Bring out a skillet pan and put it over medium heat. Add the butter and when it melts, add in the egg mixture and cook for 3 to 5 min until eggs have scrambled to the desired level.

Nutrition:

- Calories 160 kcal

- Fats 7 g

- Protein 2 g

- Carbohydrates 0 g

30. <u>Cheesy Turkey Bake</u>

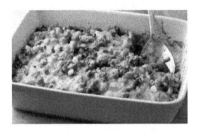

Preparation Time: 5 minutes

Cooking Time: 25 minutes

Servings: 4

Ingredients:

- 1 turkey breast, skinless, boneless, cut into strips and browned

- 2 teaspoons of olive oil

- 2 cups of almond milk

- 2 cups of cheddar cheese, shredded

- 2 eggs, whisked

- Salt and black pepper to the taste

- 1 tablespoon of chives, chopped

Directions:

1. In a bowl, mix the eggs with milk, cheese, salt, pepper, and the chives and whisk well.

2. Preheat the air fryer at 330 °F, add the oil, heat it, add the turkey pieces, and spread them well.

3. Add the egg mixture, toss a bit, and cook for 25 minutes.

4. Serve right away for breakfast.

Nutrition:

- Calories 244 kcal

- Fat 11 g

- Fiber 4 g

- Carbohydrates 5 g

- Protein 7 g

31. <u>Tomatoes and Eggs Mix</u>

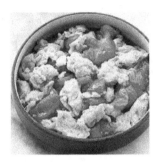

Preparation Time: 5 minutes

Cooking Time: 25 minutes

Servings: 4

Ingredients:

- 1 and 1/2 tablespoons of olive oil

- 30 ounces of canned tomatoes, chopped

- ½ pound of cheddar, shredded

- 2 tablespoons of chives, chopped

- Salt and black pepper to the taste

- 6 eggs, whisked

Directions:

1. Put the oil in the air fryer, heat it at 350 ° F, add the tomatoes, eggs, salt, and pepper, and whisk.

2. Add the cheese on top and sprinkle the chives on top.

3. Cook for around 25 minutes, divide between plates and serve for breakfast.

Nutrition:

- Calories 221 kcal

- Fat 8 g

- Fiber 3 g

- Carbohydrates 4 g

- Protein 8 g

32. Creamy Almond and Cheese Mix

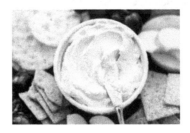

Preparation Time: 10 minutes

Cooking Time: 20 minutes

Servings: 6

Ingredients:

- 1-cup of almond milk

- Cooking spray

- 9 ounces of cream cheese, soft

- 1 cup of cheddar cheese, shredded

- 6 spring onions, chopped

- Salt and black pepper to the taste

- 6 eggs, whisked

Directions:

1. Heat up your air fryer with the oil at 350 ° F and grease it with cooking spray.

2. In a bowl, put and mixed the eggs with the rest of the ingredients, whisk well, pour and spread into the air fryer and cook everything for 20 minutes.

3. Divide everything between plates and serve.

Nutrition:

- Calories 231 kcal

- Fat 11 g

- Fiber 3 g

- Carbohydrates 5 g

- Protein 8 g

33. <u>Olives Bake</u>

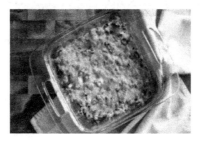

Preparation Time: 5 minutes

Cooking Time: 20 minutes

Servings: 4

Ingredients:

- 2 cups of black olives, pitted and chopped

- 4 eggs, whisked

- ¼-teaspoon of sweet paprika

- 1 tablespoon of cilantro, chopped

- ½ cup of cheddar, shredded

- A pinch of salt and black pepper Cooking spray

Directions:

1. In a bowl, put and mix the eggs with the olives and all the ingredients except the cooking spray and stir well.

2. Heat the air fryer at 350 °F; grease it with cooking spray, pour the olives and eggs mixture, spread, and cook for 20 minutes.

3. Divide between plates and serve for breakfast.

Nutrition:

- Calories 240 kcal

- Fat 14 g

- Fiber 3 g

- Carbohydrates 5 g

- Protein 8 g

CHAPTER 7. DINNER

34. Meatballs with Eggplant

Preparation Time: 15 minutes

Cooking Time: 60 minutes

Servings: 6

Ingredients:

- 1-pound of ground beef

- ½ cup of green bell pepper, chopped

- 2 medium eggplants, peeled and diced

- ½ teaspoon of minced garlic

- 1 cup of stewed tomatoes

- ½ cup of white onion, diced

- 1/3 cup of canola oil

- 1 teaspoon of lemon and pepper seasoning, salt-free

- 1 teaspoon of turmeric

- 1 teaspoon of Mrs. Dash seasoning blend

- 2 cups of water

Directions:

1. Take a large skillet pan, place it over medium heat, add oil in it, add garlic plus green bell pepper and cook within 4 minutes until sautéed.

2. Transfer green pepper mixture to a plate, set aside until needed. Then, put the eggplant pieces into the pan and cook within 4 minutes per side until browned, and when done, transfer the eggplant to a plate and set aside until needed.

3. Take a medium bowl, place beef in it, add onion, season with all the spices, stir until well combined, and then shape the batter into 30 small meatballs.

4. Place meatballs into the pan in a single layer and cook for 3 minutes, or until browned.

5. When done, place all the meatballs in the pan, add cooked bell pepper mixture in it along with eggplant, stir in water and tomatoes.

6. Simmer for 30 minutes at a low heat setting until thoroughly cooked. Serve straight away.

Nutrition:

- Calories 265 kcal Fat 18 g Protein 17 g Sodium 153 mg

- Carbohydrates 12 g Potassium 598 mg Phosphorus 193 mg

35. <u>Pepper Steak</u>

Preparation Time: 10 minutes

Cooking Time: 25minutes

Servings: 6

Ingredients:

- 3 pounds of steaks, cut into strips

- 2 cups of green bell pepper, chopped

- 1 medium white onion, peeled and minced

- 1 cup of carrots, sliced

- ½ cup of celery, chopped

- 1 package of brown gravy mix

- 2 tablespoons of olive oil

- 1 ¼ cup of water

Directions:

1. Take a large skillet pan, place it over medium-high heat, add oil and when hot, add steak strips and cook for 7 to 10 minutes, or until browned.

2. Then add all the vegetables, pour in ¼-cup of water, and cook for 8 minutes until softened, covering the pan.

3. Stir in brown gravy mix, then pour in the remaining water, switch the heat to medium heat and cook for 5 minutes until the sauce has reduced to the desired thickness. Serve straight away.

Nutrition:

- Calories 340 kcal

- Fat 340 g

- Protein 33 g

- Sodium 285 mg

- Carbohydrates 7 g

- Potassium 596 mg

- Phosphorus 338 mg

36. <u>Stuffed Peppers</u>

Preparation Time: 10 minutes

Cooking Time: 1 hour and 20 minutes

Servings: 4

Ingredients:

- ¾ pound of ground beef

- ½ cup of white onion, chopped

- 4 medium green bell peppers, destemmed and cored

- 1 tablespoon of dried parsley

- 1 ½ teaspoon of garlic powder

- 1 teaspoon of ground black pepper

- 2 cups of cooked white rice

- 3 ounces of tomato sauce, unsalted

Directions:

1. Switch on the oven, then set it to 375 °F and let it preheat. Take a medium-sized saucepan, place it over medium heat and when hot, add beef and cook for 10 minutes, or until browned.

2. Then drain the excess fat, add the remaining ingredients (except for green bell pepper), stir until combined, and simmer for 10 minutes until cooked.

3. When done, spoon the beef mixture evenly between peppers, place the peppers into a baking dish, and bake for 1 hour until cooked. Serve straight away.

Nutrition:

- Calories 264 kcal

- Fat 7 g

- Protein 20 g

- Sodium 213 mg

- Carbohydrates 28 g

- Potassium 553 mg

- Phosphorus 209 mg

37.   <u>Barley and Beef Stew</u>

Preparation Time: 10 minutes

Cooking Time: 1 hour and 15 minutes

Servings: 6

Ingredients:

- 1-pound of beef stew meat, 1 ½ inch, cubed

- 1 cup of pearl barley, soaked for 1 hour

- ½ cup of white onion, diced

- 2 medium carrots, peeled and sliced

- 1 large stalk of celery, diced

- 2 tablespoons of all-purpose white flour

- ½ teaspoon of minced garlic

- ¼ teaspoon of ground black pepper

- ½ teaspoon of salt

- 1 teaspoon of onion herb seasoning

- 2 tablespoons of canola oil

- 2 bay leaves

- 8 cups of water

Directions:

1. Place beef in a plastic bag, add flour and black pepper, seal the bag and shake well until well coated.

2. Take a large pot, place it over medium heat, add oil, and when hot, add coated beef and cook for 10 minutes until browned.

3. When done, transfer beef to a plate, add celery, onion, and garlic, cook for 2 minutes, pour in water, and bring the mixture to a boil.

4. Add beef into the boiling mixture, then switch heat to medium level, season with salt, add bay leaf and barley to the pot, stir until mixed and cook for 1 hour until cooked through, stirring every 15 minutes.

5. When done, add carrots, stir in herb seasoning, continue cooking for 1 hour and then serve.

Nutrition:

- Calories 246 kcal

- Fat 8 g

- Protein 22 g Sodium 222 mg

- Carbohydrates 21 g Potassium 369 mg

- Phosphorus 175 mg

38. <u>Chicken and Corn Soup</u>

Preparation Time: 15 minutes

Cooking Time: 60 minutes

Servings: 12

Ingredients:

- 6 ounces of flat noodles, medium-sized, cooked

- 4-pound of roasting chicken

- 10 ounces of cooked corn

- ¼ teaspoon of ground black pepper

- 1 tablespoon of parsley, chopped

- 14 cups of water

Directions:

1. Take a large pot, place it over medium heat, pour in 8 cups water, add chicken, cook within 30 to 40 minutes until the chicken has cooked, and when done, separate chicken from broth and set aside until needed.

2. Meanwhile, cook the noodles until tender, omit the salt and when cooked, drain the noodles, and set aside until required.

3. Remove fat from the chicken broth by skimming it, let the chicken cool slightly, and then cut it into bite-size pieces.

4. Take a large pot, place it over medium heat, pour in broth and the remaining water, stir in chicken, add cooked noodles and corn, stir in black pepper and parsley and simmer for 15 to 20 minutes until hot. When done, ladle soup into bowls and then serve.

Nutrition:

- Calories 222 kcal

- Fat 6 g

- Protein 25 g

- Sodium 240 mg

- Carbohydrates 17 g

- Potassium 303 mg

- Phosphorus 212 mg

39. <u>Asparagus, Chicken and Wild Rice Soup</u>

Preparation Time: 10 minutes

Cooking Time: 45 minutes

Servings: 8

Ingredients:

- 2 cups of cooked chicken

- ¾ cup of wild rice and white rice blend, cooked

- ½ cup of all-purpose white flour

- 2 cups of asparagus, diced

- 1 cup of carrots, diced

- ½ cup of white onion, diced

- 1 ½ teaspoon of minced garlic

- ½ teaspoon of salt

- ½ teaspoon of dried thyme

- ½ teaspoon of ground black pepper

- ½ teaspoon of ground nutmeg

- 1 bay leaf

- ¼ cup of unsalted butter

- ½ cup of dry vermouth

- 4 cups of chicken broth, low-sodium

- 4 cups of almond milk, unenriched, unsweetened

Directions:

1. Take a Dutch oven, place over medium heat, add the butter and when it melts, add the onion, garlic and cook it for 5 minutes or until tender

2. Then add carrots, stir in all the spices and herbs, continue cooking for 5 minutes or until carrots are tender.

3. Switch to low heat, stir in flour, continue cooking for 10 minutes, then pour in vermouth and chicken broth and whisk until combined.

4. Add chicken and asparagus, then gradually stir in milk and continue simmering for 20 minutes until cooked. When done, fold rice into the soup and then serve.

Nutrition:

- Calories 295 kcal Fat 11 g Protein 21 g

- Sodium 385 mg Carbohydrates 28 g

- Potassium 527 mg Phosphorus 252 mg

40. **Green Chili Stew**

Preparation Time: 10 minutes

Cooking Time: 10 hours and 10 minutes **Servings:** 6

Ingredients:

- 1-pound of pork chops, cubed 8 ounces of green chilies, diced

- ¾ cup of iceberg lettuce, shredded

- ½ cup of all-purpose white flour

- ¼ cup of cilantro, chopped

- ½ teaspoon of minced garlic

- 1 tablespoon of garlic powder

- 1 teaspoon of ground black pepper

- 1 tablespoon of olive oil 6 tablespoons of sour cream

- 14 ounces of chicken broth, low-sodium

- 6 flour tortillas, burrito-size

Directions:

1. Put flour in your large plastic bag, add black pepper and garlic powder, then add pork cubes. Seal the bag, then shake well until coated.

2. Take a large skillet pan, place it over medium heat, add oil and when hot, add pork pieces and cook for 10 minutes, or until browned.

3. Switch on the slow cooker, place pork in it, add garlic and chilies, pour in the broth, shut with the lid, and cook pork for 10 hours at low heat setting until tender.

4. When done, place ¾ cup of pork on the tortilla, roll it like a burrito, and serve with lettuce, cilantro, and sour cream.

Nutrition:

- Calories 420 kcal

- Fat 16 g

- Protein 25 g

- Sodium 552 mg

- Carbohydrates 44 g

- Potassium 454 mg

- Phosphorus 323 mg

CONCLUSION

Intermittent fasting is not a new direction of dieting. In fact, people have been doing it since the beginning of time. Certain fasts, such as the Ramadan fast, Lent, etc., have been practiced since ancient times. Though based on beliefs and religions, these fasts are still forms of intermittent fasts and have similar positive effects as well. Intermittent fasting basically means eating at particular times during the day and fasting for the remaining time. So, for instance, if you have your breakfast at 8:00 a.m., you are supposed to fast until 8:00 p.m. The fasting period allows your body a resting period and leads to weight loss, glucose regulation, and various other benefits.

There exist a variety of intermittent fasts. Some of them are easy to do, while some are quite difficult for beginners. Regardless of the ease of an intermittent fast, it can still be one of the most difficult things you ever do if you have never fasted before. You need to regulate your diet cycle, which can be quite a task for many. Yet, it can't be compared to the grueling fact that you need to go 'hungry' for 8-10-12 or even more hours of the day. Eating one or two meals per day and going 'hungry' for the rest is especially difficult for people with busy schedules who are often accustomed to eating anything they find whenever they get the time. Such people avoid doing intermittent fasting because they believe that they cannot stick to the diet or will go hungry.

CPSIA information can be obtained
at www.ICGtesting.com
Printed in the USA
BVHW092304140621
609528BV00010B/1489

9 781803 008882